WEIGHT LOSS INSPIRATION

How to Lose Weight Naturally, Without Quitting in the Middle

AMINE SALHI

TABLE OF CONTENTS

CHAPTER 1

WHY LOVE?

How are love and weight loss connected? Are they even? These are the questions that one might choose to ask herself. Astonished as we are by this unexpected link, something deep within tells us that there is a direct link between the two. Love/self-love and being fulfilled with one's body — these are two sides of one coin. Whether we like it or not, if we do not love ourselves, it is highly unlikely that we will manage to create the body of our dreams. By create, I am note talking about excruciating exercise routines and diets that leave one feeling depleted emotionally. I am talking about a body that one feels comfortable in, a body that is cozy. Just like a comfortable and spacious house, a healthy body is a good place to live in.

However, it is not always easy to reach this state of goodness. At times, it might be so much easier to squeeze oneself into a paradigm of dieting, weight loss, and other harsh or not so harsh ways for managing one's weight (and body image). Yet, before we jump into the topic of weight loss, we should most certainly deconstruct the very concept of body image. What are our bodies like? How do we learn to perceive these beautiful machines? Who teaches us the most crucial lessons of self-perception? How do we come to despise ourselves? While "despise" might sound like a very strong word, in effect, this is often how many of us perceive our bodies or certain parts of it.

In my opinion, we are born beautiful and healthy and strong. However, when we come into contact with society, we adopt a certain perception of ourselves, our characters and our bodies, that is very far from the truth. Oftentimes, we develop a "false" self that is meant to satisfy everyone but us. This false self might even become our primary self, the one we turn to for advice and reassurance. Yet, there is one "small" problem. This false self is not on our side. Since it was constructed by society and its various false postulates, it is unlikely that this false self will show any compassion or love for our true, authentic selves. Stay with me here. This is one of the most important parts in this book. If you get this, the rest will come to you like a breeze.

We go about life with a false sense of self, tending to believe that in order to be lovable, we must behave a certain way, look a certain way, etc. But nothing could be farther from the truth. We cannot live from the shell. It has no energy. To tap into that inner source of love and life, we must go deep within ourselves, find that true, authentic self, and start living from it. This is a process that is filled with fear. Much fear. Very much fear. However, if you manage this process well, sooner or later, your body, spirit, and psyche will be integrated to form a single unit. They will become One. It is from this state of oneness that any lasting and true change can come. Whether this be change in one's mind, one's emotional realm, one's spiritual world, or one's body.

So where do we start? Let's take a close look.

CHAPTER 2

TELL YOURSELF THE TRUTH (AND ONLY THE TRUTH)

What do you love about your body? What do you hate about your body? What are you embarrassed of? Answer each of these questions in written form and only then continue reading. Because if you do not have an honest conversation with yourself, it is unlikely that you will be able to really grasp the message of this book. Now that you have answered each of these questions, get down to these next few inquiries turned inward: How did you come to love these parts of yourself? How did you come to hate these other parts of yourself? Was it a certain situation or a set of situations that made you experience these feelings? Who was a part of this situation? How did your body image fluctuate as a result of these experiences? As you move along answering these questions, pay attention to your feelings, your bodily sensations, your thoughts, and write them down as well. Can you hear your body trying to talk to you? Can you hear it trying to open up that box of old memories that you have locked up? The memories that have made you into the person you are today. Certainly, all this might feel slightly like a therapeutic session, and it is, in a way. I call this self-therapy. It can be as effective and helpful as talking to a psychotherapist. While self-therapy and therapy do not exclude each other, every one of us, at a certain point, comes to the realization that we cannot depend on other people for answering those questions which we must answer ourselves. Others cannot do our inner work for us.

Below, I will mention a rather long list of questions that you should try to answer when left all to yourself in a tranquil state of mind. If you doubt a certain answer, move further and return to this question or set of questions the next day. I also suggest that you have a separate notebook for this work, not to confuse it with your other written records. What is more, it might help to readdress these questions once in a while, since your answers might change, because you, as a human being, undergo constant changes and shifts.

When reading these questions, write down whatever first comes to mind. It is very important not to mentally filter your answers, as the first replies are the most honest ones.

Here it goes.

1. Do you love yourself?

2. What is it that you love most?

3. What is it that you love least?

4. If you could change any two things about yourself, what would they be?

5. What would you leave as it is (never changing it, since you love these things about yourself so much)?

6. What about your body? What are your favorite body parts? Least favorite?

7. Who is your closest friend? Closest relative?

8. Are you in a conflicting relationship with someone at present? Who? Why?

9. If you could change this, would you? How?

10. How is this impacting your feelings toward yourself?

11. How are these feelings impacting your body image?

12. Have you ever thought about plastic surgery?

13. What are your favorite sports (list five)?

14. How often do you engage in exercise?

15. How many times a day do you think negatively about your body? *Get down to it and keep count!

16. Write down these negative thoughts?

17. What are your positive thoughts about your body?

18. Undress yourself and stand in front of the mirror. Look at your body and write down the 10 things you love and 10 things you do not like about your body. You can change the number if you do not feel comfortable with 10.

19. Finally, write down any thoughts and fantasies that you might have had when answering these questions. Did you discover anything new about yourself? Were you already aware of these inner processes prior to doing the exercise?

I hope you had fun! You might ask why I started the chapter by asking questions, if there was a list of questions to be found in the end of this chapter. First and foremost, because I wanted you to have a small warm up session that would get you thinking about complex and difficult topics. Just like our bodies, our brains need to be warmed up properly and constantly, before we engage in a fully fledged exercise routine.

CHAPTER 3

START WITH THE MIND, ALWAYS

We have already started, haven't we? If you answered all of the abovementioned questions, you can move on with this chapter. If not, please, return to the latter chapter and finish up those questions. It is crucial that you establish a strong and lasting bond with yourself. In fact, this is the only way to experiencing true bliss, success, and love in your life. What do you want? Where are you heading?

How does weight loss even fit within all of these categories. My personal journey of weight loss which lasted for 20 years taught me one important lesson: if you are enemies with your body, you will not make it. You have to make friends with your body. Once and forever. There is nothing more tempting that running off and away from yourself, while absorbing others' perception of you and adopting goals that are not your own. However, this is not the right path. It is the wrong path, which will lead you to years and years of suffering and pain.

When you practice weight loss without your mind truly involved, without being truly frank with yourself, you will end up in a dark place. Like I did. One moment you feel like you have made a huge leap in terms of weight loss, another moment, you are fighting those demons again. The demons that tell you that despite all your efforts, you are just not good enough (yes, because you ate that second muffin). Just look at this example with a clear head and understand: this is not healthy. And you probably know it. So how do you establish a truly healthy relationship with yourself and your body? Listen. Listen to yourself. Listen to your body. Listen to your emotions.

And ask yourself: why do I eat? Is it because of hunger? Is it emotional eating? What is it? What stands behind my food habits? Huh. Not an easy one. I must tell you, as a nutritionist and someone who "fought" with my body for decades, we often eat emotionally. This is why weight loss needs to involve two realms: the body and the mind. And the mind comes first. In fact, I advise that aside from exercise and healthy eating, you engage in some kind of counseling and/or coaching to work through the issues that you were able to recognize in the prior chapter. Some people can work through these issues by themselves via meditation, yoga, journaling. Yet others, like me, need outside help. Please, do not hesitate to turn to a specialist who will help you to work through your body image issues. However, since you are holding this book here and now, I will do my best to share my experience with you and maybe it will help you to make that one crucial leap forward.

CHAPTER 4

ON TO THE BODY

Why is it that we decide to go against our bodies at one point or another? By "go against" I mean all the self-loathing and self-hate that modern-day culture is filled with when it comes to our bodies. This is often difficult to recognize, however, this hate is concealed in the smallest details: the way we look after our bodies, the way we take care of them, how we do all of these things… Just look at the various advertisements that surround us on a daily basis. We are convinced that we should look better, smell better, dress better, etc. It is like we are never enough. In fact, we live in a "not enough" culture and we are immersed in this culture from a very early age. Because of this, we start to believe in a false story about ourselves, about our bodies.

In fact, have you ever thought about why so many people in our time have various kinds of mental illnesses (disorders)? In my opinion and based on my experience, this happens because of a disconnect between the body and the mind. We stop feeling ourselves (our own feelings) and literally "jump" out of our bodies, trying to become somebody else.

When we are very young, our parents and society instils numerous false beliefs in us. These false beliefs then guide how we feel about ourselves. However, in this book, what I am trying to teach you is to listen to your body. Listen to it. Oh, yes. It has a voice. It has its own tastes. You should never stop listening to it and if you did, a long time ago, then now is the time to start listening to it. At this point, I would like to introduce to you the idea of **intuitive** eating. What is this? Hah, it's not that easy to grasp, but you will manage if you try.

Below, I present a series of tips that you might want to try out.

Tip 1: When you get up in the morning, ask yourself what is the first thing that you want to eat. And when you answer this question, make sure that you are relaxed and focusing on your bodily sensations. Does your body want water? Warm water? Cold water? Water with lemon? Do you want to eat right away or do you feel repulsed at the very thought of food and need some time to get hungry?

Tip 2: Throughout the day, when you are about to eat something that is familiar, ask yourself again and again: "Do I want this?" Or are you eating this food just to fill a certain emotional gap in your psyche? Oftentimes, we eat something because we feel down, or sad, or angry (the range of emotions can go on and on).

Tip 3: Give yourself time to process the food that you are eating. First, mentally. Then, physically. By mental processing I mean coming in touch with your food, being aware of your wishes and fulfilling them, while avoiding overeating. This means imagining first that you are eating something and only then deciding whether you want to eat this food in reality. Oftentimes, it happens so that we do not actually want to eat; if you look at your emotions more closely, it might turn out that you are not hungry, but rather, you are linking a certain emotion to a given food (and in an attempt to experience or avoid experiencing this emotion you are drawn toward that food). However, if you realize that the food you are thinking of is what you actually want to consume, try to do this slowly, without hustle and bustle. Concentrate on your eating process. Chew slowly. Enjoy. It is crucial that you enjoy your meal or snack.

Tip 4: Make a top 10 list of the foods that you love and next to each position write down an emotion that is linked to this specific food. This way, unconscious habits will be made conscious. For instance, when I made my list, I realized that chocolate was linked to happiness in my case. As for snacks such as cookies and crackers, I consumed that as "munchies" when I was procrastinating. In fact, it is very interesting to explore why and how you consume certain foods. You can write down more than 10 foods, yet 10 is minimum.

CHAPTER 5

WHAT DO YOU LOVE?

You might be surprised by the fact that such a broad question is presented as the title of this chapter. However, do not be surprised. Love and weight loss are directly linked. This is something that we have never been told before. In fact, we are told by society and advertisements that only upon reaching a certain weight/body goal will we feel love for our bodies. Yet, I believe that the cause-effect link is absolutely the opposite. First, we come to a place of love within us and only from that place can we actually change something about our bodies. Here, I am talking about lasting, conscious change. Change that will stick with us in time.

The problem with dieting and other weight loss techniques is that they give one a temporary result. If not supported by the right philosophy, these efforts will often lead to results that wane sooner or later. The extra pounds are back within months or less, the motivation dies out, and so on. Why and when does this happen? This happens when an individual strives toward weight loss without a solid basis, which is love. Self-love. Thus, in order to lose weight wisely and for long, one must address the body from a place of love. If we despise our bodies, it is unlikely that we will do them good.

Hating something and trying to change it through self-abuse (strict dieting and stringent exercise schedules) will not bring you to a "happier place."

What I am trying to show here, in this chapter, is that happiness, love, and weight loss are all part of a single cocktail. A cocktail called life. We live in a time when problems should be approached holistically. Today, humanity has come to a new level of understanding — understanding the human body, the human journey, and our human reality. "Easy" solutions no longer work. Their results are short-term. However, for long-term changes and outcomes, we have to go deeper within ourselves. This "deep" diving is essential to a fulfilling and long life.

Now that I have discussed in detail the philosophy of weight loss, I would like to move on to a more thorough exploration of the daily tips and practices that could help one to start-off on a journey of weight loss and self-love.

CHAPTER 6

DAILY TIPS AND PRACTICES

Exercise

Let's start with the body. Ask yourself some crucial questions. These questions concern your daily routine and physical activity. Do you practice sports and exercise on a daily basis? How many times a week do you engage in active physical activity? Walking? Dancing? Swimming? Etc. Make a list of the days of the week, from Monday to Sunday, and record over a period of two weeks your activity schedules. If you have a smart watch or special apps on your phone, you can use those to make a record of all your physical activities.

Do you engage in some kind of a physical activity for at least 30 minutes per day? This is the minimum. By physical activity, I mean a brisk walk in the park, a jog, a series of stretching or yoga exercises. What are your favorite sports? Make a list of three and make sure to include these sports in your weekly schedule. Below, I present an example of a schedule that works for me. Your task is to come up with your own routine that you will find pleasurable.

Monday

30-minute walk in the park

Tuesday

1-hour workout at the gym

Wednesday

40 minutes of yoga before work in the morning

Thursday

45-minute jog in the park

Friday

40-minute swim

Saturday

1-hour dance class

Sunday

1-hour walk in the park

You see, if you are trying to engage in various kinds of exercise that you despise, you are not doing yourself good. You have to really truly look forward to that workout, walk, dance class, or whatever else it is you choose to practice. If you feel depleted after your workout, you are destroying your health (mental and physical), little by little, since you are doing something that you basically hate. Remember, we talked about self-love and the importance of engaging in weight loss from a place of love? If you engage in an exercise routine that leaves you feeling unhappy, sooner or later you will drop this routine. However, if you find the right kind of physical activity (one that suits you), you will feel refreshed and enlivened after your work out. Do not deprive yourself of the wonderful opportunity to feel that positive after-effect of exercise. Thus, I hope you have "heard" the message that this chapter conveys: exercise has to make you happy. Certainly, at times, you might not feel like taking that morning walk. But slight resistance is alright, as long as it does not feel like moving against a brick wall of resistance. In the end, you will recognize your kind of physical activity via your sensations after the class or exercise session is over.

Ask yourself the following list of questions after each of your exercise sessions:

- Do I feel enlivened?

- Do I feel energized?

- Would I like to repeat what I just did some days later?

- Did I derive pleasure from the process?

- Do I feel emotionally depleted or fulfilled?

- Do I feel happy that I engaged in this physical activity?

- What would I change about this physical activity to make it even better? (Examples could be: create a special playlist to accompany me during the exercise session; practice during a different time throughout the day, when I feel more energized).

What I am trying to demonstrate here is that you have to make your exercise schedule most convenient for you. It has to suit you and your needs, first and foremost. Exercise is not a battle with your body. It is a series of small to medium efforts that, in the end, bring you to the right destination. This destination is a healthy and vivacious body, as well as a positive, focused mind. It is no secret that workouts help to boost our mental processes. Any kind of physical activity can be perceived as a kind of meditation. It helps to structure our thinking and free ourselves from unneeded emotional states. You will certainly experience a kind of emotional cleansing as a result of regular physical activity.

<u>Diet</u>

Next, I would like to offer some nice diet tips that will help you to keep your energy levels high. Based on my experience and all that I have studied about various kinds of diets, it is crucial that you reduce the amount of processed foods to an absolute minimum. By processed foods I mean pre-prepared meals that you can find in a supermarket. These meals might seem like a convenient solution, yet, at the end of the day, they contain many sugars and saturated fats, as well as carbs, that will not do your body good. Try to focus more on fruits and vegetables. In fact, I advise you to follow the recommendations offered by the food pyramid, while placing a slightly heavier emphasis on the consumption of fruits/vegetables. Below, I offer my own interpretation of the food pyramid, suggesting the precise number of servings of each kind of food that should be consumed on a daily basis.

1. Fruits/vegetables: 7-8 servings per day.

2. Cereals, rice, pasta: 7-8 servings per day.

3. Milk Products: 2 servings per day.

4. Fish: 1-2 servings per day.

5. Meat: 3 servings per week.

6. Sweets (containing sugars), fats: 2-3 servings per week, yet it is best to exclude such foods.

One of the most crucial tips that I would like to give you is to remove all processed sugars from your diet. If this is too difficult to do, try reducing such foods to a maximum of 2 to 3 servings per week. This means getting rid of all those salty, fatty, and sugary snacks and substituting them with healthy snacks.

Below, I suggest some ideas of healthy snacks that you might find useful:

- carrot/celery sticks;

- apple;

- banana;

- exotic fruits (passion fruit, mango, etc.);

- whole grain crackers;

- dried fruit;

- nuts (almonds, cashew, walnut, etc.);

- smoothies;

- freshly squeezed juices.

You are welcome to complement this list with other ideas of snacks that you find both tasty and healthy. Overall, the goal of this chapter is to emphasize that you should eat foods that have undergone minimum processing. Excluding fried foods from your diet is an absolute must. Of course, a once-per-month McDonalds meal will not kill you. However, when you remove fried and processed foods from your diet, within a week or two you will notice one interesting phenomenon — after a period of excessive craving comes another period, that of indifference. Yes, you will no longer look at junk food with the longing of an addict, since your body will get used to healthier options, driving pleasure from these foods vs. the sugary/fatty foods you used to soothe yourself. What is more, at a certain point, you will wonder why you found junk food so appealing. The smell, the look of it will no longer trigger your senses. But, please, keep in mind that the first few weeks are the most difficult. You have to come prepared and equipped.

How can you equip yourself to resist all those cravings? Make a list of all the healthy foods and put it on your fridge (and have a copy of it in your phone if you tend to eat out often). When you feel hungry, look at this list and make a choice. In fact, I suggest that you make a list of the healthy meals that you choose from on a regular basis. For instance, it would be best if you list 10 options of healthy breakfast, lunch, and dinner (as well as snacks). This way, you will have a total of 10 options to choose from on a regular basis. However, all of these options must be qualified as healthy. They should be high in fiber, low-sugar, low-fat, whole grain, fresh, and not processed (or minimum processing). As for the methods of preparation, I suggest that you prepare your foods via steaming/boiling or baking. These are the healthiest options. Also, use as little butter and processed fats as possible. When you need to use oil, stick to fresh-pressed, unprocessed oils.

One thing that we have not touched upon is water. You have to drink a lot of water on a daily basis. I am sure you have heard this many times, yet we often underestimate the importance of this advice (and, believe me, it is highly important!). At least 2 liters of water daily. Do whatever it takes you to make sure that you drink this much (or more) water on a daily basis.

How can you increase your water consumption?

- Carry around a water bottle with you; refill it constantly.

- Drink a glass of water (or two!) in the morning.

- Drink one glass of water (200 milliliters) every 1-1.5 hours.

- Make sure that you drink water at least 30 minutes before a meal or 1 hour after. It is best not to mix food and water.

If you stick to these tips, I am more than sure that you will see some tremendous and lasting changes taking place within 3 weeks of time. What are they? A more fit and beautiful body. What is most important, you are bound to see your energy levels rise (immensely). Also, if you have problems with falling or staying asleep at night, these changes in your diet and physical activity levels will help you to sleep better. As a matter of fact, nothing was said about sleep above, and sleep is one of the most important aspects of health. Not sleeping enough has a toll on your body. It leaves you depleted and can negatively impact your mood. Thus, it is highly important that you get those 8 hours of sleep per night to avoid long-term damage to your body and mind.

CHAPTER 7

THERE IS NO ONE PILL TO SWALLOW

When it comes to weight loss, many of us want results, immediate results. We are not willing to invest the time and efforts that are so crucial for introducing lasting change. In order to see lasting changes come into our lives, we need to drop the "all or nothing" approach and to opt for the "step-by-step" one instead. Now, you might find my next statement slightly astonishing, yet it is as it is. It is not about weight loss, after all. It is about You and how you see yourself. About self-acceptance. And what this book is trying to teach you is that **self-acceptance** is a long and difficult path. It takes time, it takes practice, it takes wit, knowledge, and patience!

Whether you need to lose weight in order to improve your health or you have been merely infected with the idea that you need to lose weight, the issue of weight somehow bothers you. It is my aim and responsibility to teach you to distinguish between weight loss that is timely, important, and needed, and the infectious idea of weight loss that you might have absorbed through social media and other media channels. However, if you are overweight (I am talking about serious extra weight that needs to be reduced for health purposes), you are most probably more than aware of this fact. In this case, you need to take it slowly and to start with self-love.

A position of self-loathing will not take you anywhere. Moreover, if you try to cling on to a weight loss program that does not suit you, this will only make things worse. All of the universal, "swallow this pill and you will be cured" kind of approaches NEVER work. Never. And this is the first and last time that I am writing something in caps lock mode in this book. Because I want to make it absolutely clear to you: you simply must know where to start. Like in a board game, you need to get back to point one and prioritize. Based on these priorities, you draw up a map. Your own map. Don't try taking another person's map, as it will not work for you. I assure you. So, what should you take into account when putting this map together? These four points:

1. The position of Self-Love vs. self-hate.

2. Stay true to your inner core and values.

3. Do everything with grace and love.

4. Give yourself time. Time.

I suggest that you start out by asking yourself the following questions (on paper):

- Why do I want to lose weight?

- Which actions am I ready to undertake to reach my goal?

- How much weight do I want to lose?

- What is the time period for this goal?

- How will I change my diet? (Draw up the lists that were discussed prior).

- Which kinds of exercises will I be engaging in on a daily basis?

- How do I ensure that I get enough sleep on a daily basis?

As you move along, you might think of your own questions that I forgot to mention here. This is a good sign. It means that your brain is actively working to solve the issue at hand. In fact, your intuition is one of the best tools that will help you out a lot on your weight loss journey. Tune into it. It will tell you when you are overdoing it and when you are simply being a lazy bum. However, make sure that you are listening to your intuition and not some other voice in your head. Among the "false" voices that might pretend to be "intuition" you might find: the tyrant, the victim, the lazy bum. The tyrant will force you to overdo it over and over again, to the point where your weight loss journey turns into hell. An obsession. Do not let this happen. This is why you need to have a nice, comfortable plan and stick to it 24/7. The victim usually comes along with the tyrant; this voice will whine in a tiresome and constant fashion, telling you that you need to stop the self-torture (that is, weight loss gone bad). Finally, the lazy bum is that "couch" voice that just tells you to leave things as they are.

Sure, you can, but only if you agree with the idea that nothing will budge, move, or change until you roll up your sleeves and do something. If you are "ok" with your body and the life you are living now, then this book is not really for you. However, if you have made it your goal to lose weight and attain a healthy, comfortable number on your scale, please, read on. And do not listen to the lazy bum who is trying to make you give up.

CHAPTER 8

THE FOCAL POINT — SELF-CARE

I know, we have already talked about this many, many times in this book. However, I believe that this is a topic that has no beginning and no end. It is an endlessly important and grasping topic. That of self-care. Self-love. And all that comes with these two concepts. At the end of the day, weight loss should be a part of self-care. It should be imbued with elements of self-care. There is no other way of losing weight, actually. Here, I am talking about losing weight in a way that is healthy for one's body and psyche.

The objective of weight loss is one's wellbeing. Being liked by others more cannot be an objective of weight loss. Being sexier, more lovable, landing the job of one's dreams, etc. All this cannot and should not guide one's weight loss efforts. In fact, weight loss should be viewed as an integral part of one's self-care plan, if the individual is overweight. Now, when the individual's weight is normal and weight loss is no longer an objective, self-care (which includes exercising and healthy eating) should remain a top priority, with weight loss being omitted from the list of goals.

In order to dissipate the confusion that you might feel after reading the abovementioned paragraph, I would like to bring up my own example. When I started my weight loss journey, I was distraught. I felt miserable and unable to stick to all those promises that I made. I would regularly skip my workouts and have cheat meals. However, at one point I realized that the exercise schedule was too stringent and consisted of activities that I, honestly, disliked. Moreover, the diet was suggested by my nutritionist without taking into account my likes and dislikes. Basically, I was trying to adopt a lifestyle that was not my own. I was not listening to my heart, body, and soul. At all. Thus, my weight loss routine was not coming from a place of self-care, but rather from a place of "I don't like myself as I am" or we could also call it a place of self-loathing. A bad place to start off such an important transformational journey.

It took me ten years to realize this! Much time. Too much time. However, the upside of this struggle is that today I can share my experience with those who are just about to start their weight loss journeys. They can omit those mistakes which I so ruthlessly made. This is exactly why this chapter refers to self-care as the focal point of weight loss.

CHAPTER 9

RELATIONSHIPS WITH OTHERS

We often underestimate the power that others have over us. When we start any journey, it is highly important how others perceive our efforts. Do they support us? Do they laugh at us? In fact, finding a support group is a crucial part of success. This support group can include the following people: those assisting you on your weight loss journey (nutritionist, trainer), you family, friends, and other people who are struggling with extra weight. You can add to the list whomever you like. What truly matters is the relationships that you have with these people.

Since we are social beings, our relationships with others substantially impact how we view ourselves and the surrounding reality. Below, I would like to share a personal story that significantly influenced me on my weight loss path. It concerns the support that I found on my way. This support was crucial to me and my goal-attainment.

When I began my weight loss journey, I met some brilliant people on the way. They were talented, bright, and motivated. Some of them were also struggling with weight loss issues. Others, had overcome their problems and were willing to help others. Among them were people who attended various sports/exercise classes together with me. There were coaches and nutritionists who, at one point in their lives, also battled extra weight. Each one of them had their own, unique approach to weight loss. Their own, unique experience. As I mentioned above, for a decade, I tried adapting these various approaches. However, nothing really worked 100 percent. I felt like I was constantly trying to live someone else's life. At one point, a coach whom I met 10 years into my weight loss journey told me, "Stop following all these programs in an all-or-nothing kind of way. You have to find your own path. When the weight loss journey will no longer feel like a battle." And this was one of the most valuable pieces of advice ever received. From that point on, I decided that I would come up with my own theory of weight loss.

In fact, it was then that I took up meditation and onlyat that point did my weight loss journey really start. Following each of my daily meditation sessions (that lasted for 30 minutes), I was full of ideas and inspiration. I transferred these ideas on paper. In about a year or so, I had a pocketful of observations (inner and outer), contemplations, and ideas. Surely, all that led me to this state (my prior journey) was necessary and important. It gave me important food for thought. However, I had to find my own path. My own structure. And, surprisingly, it was not about a step-by-step kind of approach where you stick to a certain structure while often denying your inner states and feelings.

My philosophy of weight loss is different because I urge my clients to think outside of the box: to absorb information and then process it in a rather unique way, creating a program for themselves that will work. I advocate for weight loss approaches that are based on the notions of self-love and self-care. At the same time, it is crucial that we establish meaningful connections with others who are also undertaking this journey. Yet, not only these people. There can also be those who have never encountered an issue such as extra weight (here, I am talking about obesity issues), yet they are willing to support us on our journeys. These people are to be treasured.

As was already mentioned above, we are social beings. We subconsciously seek connection with others. This is only normal. And when we are undertaking a difficult and complex path in life, these people become more important than ever. Then, there will also be those who do not support us. Those who will make us feel less than perfect. I am talking about toxic people and toxic relationships here. In fact, such relationships can often be one of the root causes of our health issues (obesity included). It is essential that you tell yourself (and others) the truth, shying away from relationships that do not give you anything and simply take away your resources. Relationships are about mutual exchange and support! Please, remember this. It is impossible to be happy and healthy if you remain a part of something that is ultimately unhealthy.

Before I move on to the next chapter, I would like to share another personal story that had a great impact on my life. I was in a long-term relationship that was drawing much energy from me. Yet, I had gotten so used to this that I did not even notice it. Though, subconsciously, I was aware of this. I repressed my discomfort and, as a result, my body was suffering. When I took up therapy (which lasted for about two years), I made a conscious choice to honestly admit all those issues that I had been hiding from. Eventually, I decided to leave my partner in order to pursue a more fulfilling and happy life. With time, I met another person who treated me with respect, dignity, and love. Honestly, my weight loss journey went only upward from there. When I was out of my toxic relationship, I was astonished at the very thought that I had tolerated such treatment and emotional abuse for so long. Moreover, I realized that my body was carrying all of the heaviness from these toxic interactions. This heaviness was not only emotional, yet also physical.

Thus, I encourage you to closely examine not only your relationship with yourself, but also your relationships with others. Sometimes, our relationships with others can urge us to treat ourselves better. Other times, these relationships cause us to diminish ourselves; such kinds of relationships stomp on our human dignity and this is outright unacceptable. You cannot love yourself while remaining in relationships with humans who do not love you for who your are or respect you. Self-love is a two-way street. It comes from within, yet it also comes from the outside (based on how others treat us). Our identities are shaped via our interactions with others. To be 100 percent honest with ourselves, we must examine these interactions from up-close and more than once.

CHAPTER 10

INTEGRATE

Integrating the various pieces of knowledge that you acquire along the way is a must. First and foremost, you need to give yourself time. As was mentioned earlier, do not look for an easy solution or a one-fits-all kind of approach. Study the topic, gather knowledge, and integrate this information into a system, a structure that fits you. This will take time. When dealing with a serious issue such as obesity, it would be self-deceit and pretense to state that this issue is easy to solve. It is not. There are hundreds of "recipes" for weight loss. Some of them work, others do not. Have you ever asked yourself "why"? Not because these "recipes" are good or bad, but rather because they fit some, yet not others. It is all about the right fit.

Yet, in this book, I take you one step further. I want to motivate you to sew your own clothes, instead of buying something that is "all ready." To create your own approach, your own program, solution, etc. To integrate all that you already know and all that you will find out as you move along your own, unique path. Integrate. Is the key word here. As you have probably realized by now, the aim of this book is not to give you yet another pre-prepared, one-for-all kind of solution. But to give you that one, crucial push, that motivating push, which will urge you to find your own solution. Sure thing, this book offers some brief tips. However, they are complementary material. The most crucial aspect of this book is the idea that lies at its core.

Please, do your best to absorb this idea, to think it over, to contemplate about it. My aim is to help you establish a stronger bond with yourself. To hear your inner voice and accept all those parts of yourself which you might have been hiding. Some of these parts are less than pretty, but if you do not integrate them into the general framework (your life journey), you will encounter endless setbacks. Because when you are acting from a fragmented space, a fragmented sense of self, it is likely that those other parts (the repressed and rejected ones) will sabotage your journey, until you accept and integrate them.

It is easier said than done. I sure know this as a fact. However, aside from motivation, this book offers you an outline that you can use to further draw your map. In this outline you will find questions such as:

- What do I love?

- What do I treasure in life?

- What are my goals in life?

- Where am I heading?

And on to the more specific ones:

- Why do I need to lose weight?

- What are my specific goals when it comes to losing weight?

- What will I do when I have attained my goal?

As you move along, answering these questions (from the more general ones, to the more specific ones), you will feel how the various parts of you are integrated into a single whole. You need to learn to look both outward and inward, close-up and from afar. Such is the complexity of human life, the human journey.

Whether we are battling extra weight, trying to find a good job, or locking for a long-term partner to build a romantic relationship with... Each of these goals requires substantial inner work and efforts. We have to be willing to do the psychological work that comes along with goal-attainment. To integrate the micro and macro levels

CHAPTER 11

BECOME YOUR OWN GURU

Though this book offers many suggestions and tips, they are only options that you might or might not choose from. The main aim of this book was to show you that you and only you are the master of your life, body, and soul. You are the one who makes the choice. Not me. Not your nutritionist, trainer, or any other person who is assisting you in your healing and weight loss journey. You see, weight loss is always about healing. Whether you are dealing with actual obesity or an eating disorder, there is always a mental health issue that stands behind these problems.

Our relationships with food always resemble our relationships with ourselves. Each and every person has certain projections that he/she places on food. These projections can be both positive and negative. What is food to you? Is it about satisfying your physical hunger, emotional hunger, or something else? How often do you feel guilty if you satisfy your hunger a certain way? As a matter of fact, what are the key emotions that accompany your food consumption process? These are just a few questions that you might want to answer. Yet, the main goal of this book and the various pieces of advice that it offers is to get you back on track, your own track, of knowing your body (and psyche) better. You literally have to become your own guru, instead of looking for outside "gurus" who will tell you what to do. Since every human being is unique, there is no one solution for all. In fact, I urge you to find your own path, your own solution, and to stick to it, no matter what.

One last exercise that I would like to offer in this book is called "Tune into your heart." Sit down, relax, make 10 deep breaths. Then, continue reading. Imagine yourself 10 years from now. Where are you living? How do you look like? Imagine yourself standing in front of a mirror, naked. How is your body different from the one you have now? Is it the same? Is it more fit? Chubbier? Can you envision this body of the future? Do you find this process difficult? After you have answered these questions, move on to the next phase of the exercise. Imagine yourself 5 years from now. Is this image somehow different from the above one? From the body you have today? Finally, imagine how you will look a year from now.

You can carry out this exercise with eyes open or closed. It does not matter — however you find it more convenient. However, make sure to tap into the vivid imagery, the sensations, the vision. After you have finished with the three abovementioned visualizations, walk up to the mirror. Undress yourself. Look at your body, with love, devotion, and kindness. And, looking yourself in the eyes, say the following words: "You are not perfect. I am not perfect. We are not perfect. And we will never be. However, I love you. Just as you are. Here and now. And I will do my very best to take good care of you."

* * *

You see, self-love is never about loathing, or hating, or abusing your body to make it look like that model from the cover of Cosmopolitan. You have to go deeper. Further. Farther. Beyond the weight loss issue. Sometimes, weight is an issue. Yet, other times, it is an issue that lives in our heads (and only there). And the ultimate goal is to free oneself from these misconceptions and to start truly caring for our bodies via exercise, healthy eating, meditation, and any other self-care techniques that you find appealing.

In the end, you body will take the shape that is most natural for it. And your task is to love this shape, no matter how large or small. You must learn to tell yourself regularly, "I Am Enough."

And, please, remember that you are.

CHAPTER 12

THE PLAN

The goal of this chapter is to put everything together: all of the prior information. It is crucial to synthesize the information that was presented in prior chapters so that you will find it accessible and comprehensible.

Please, pick up a pen and your weight loss journal/notebook and answer these final questions. I know that you have answered some of these questions (or similar questions) in the prior chapters. At this point, consider those exercises as a warm up that was meant to prepare you for the final leap: your final plan. Let's go!

My Plan:

1. What is your motivation for weight loss?

2. Outline the time period and specific weight that you are planning to lose. *Tip: please, do not set numbers that are too large; it is best to give yourself more time in order to make the transition more gradual.

3. What are the diverse types of exercises that you are willing to engage in on your weight loss journey?

4. How much time per day are you willing to dedicate to physical activity (on a daily basis)?

5. Draw a map of your exercise plan (make a weekly plan every Sunday night that you will follow during the upcoming week). It should list days from Monday to Sunday, mentioning the specific time period that you are planning to dedicate to your physical activity sessions.

6. Do the same thing for your meals and snacks. Yet, before you do this, return to the list of healthy meals that you made as you read one of the prior chapters. If you did not do this, do it now! Then, just like you did with exercise sessions, make a weekly plan of the meals that you will eat from Monday to Sunday (breakfast, morning snack, lunch, afternoon snack, and dinner) every Sunday night. Follow through! *Tip: if one night you feel like you would rather switch to another healthy meal from your list of "healthy meals," don't hesitate. As long as you stick to unprocessed, healthy, natural foods in your diet.

7. Spiritual support. What are you going to do on a daily basis to make sure that you remain in touch with your emotional world? Mediation? Journaling? Therapy? You need to dedicate at least 30 (or more) minutes per day to this. Make a list of the "small" things that you are going to do on a daily basis to meet your spiritual needs. What will it be? 30 minutes of morning mediation and a therapeutic session every other week? Yoga? Daily journaling? Come up with this plan every Sunday night.

8. Relationship with self. You need to reexamine your relationships with yourself. This can be done via the various methods mentioned in the prior point. Also, this entails being self-aware and conscious of one's goals and motivations.

9. Relationships with others. You should also reexamine your relationships with others. Are they making you happy? Who do you want to keep in your life? Is there someone that you need to let go of, yet you have been afraid to do this? Are there any toxic relationships that need to be severed? Who are the people you treasure most? What is it that they give you (or you give them) which makes these relationships so valuable? Make a list of all those people you love and treasure — the relationships you want to hold on to. Make a list of all those relationships that you are not sure of. Why? What are your doubts about? Finally, make a list of all those relationships that you certainly want to end. Examine your feelings more closely and all of the "why's."

10. Make sure to get 8 hours of sleep per night. This is essential to your health and wellbeing. If you are feeling depleted and lack energy, it is unlikely that you will muster the will to follow through with your abovementioned goals.

11. Drink at least 2 liters of clear, non-sparkling water per day. As was suggested earlier in this book, you can drink a glass of water every 1-1.5 hours. This way, you will make sure to consume the recommended amount of water on a daily basis.

12. Hobbies. Since I am proposing a holistic approach to weight loss (one that will bring your life to a completely new level), I urge you to make a list of all those things that help you to release stress and raise your endorphin level. And, remember, happiness is conducive to weight loss. I am talking about pure happiness, not the kind of happiness induced by a doughnut. :)

13. Support group. Though relationships were mentioned above, here, I am talking about a support group that will be with you on your weight loss journey. You need to find at least five people who will become your support group. Maybe, it is your nutritionist, your coach, your friend who is also losing weight, etc. Make a list of these people and how you connect with them.

Summing up.

Thus, based on all of the mentioned points, you need to make sure to come up with an exercise/diet/spiritual plan for every single week. Make a list of all those things that you will commit to daily and follow through. The fun part is that each week you can try something new and innovate with your plan. This will help you to stay motivated and energized.

Also, do not aim too high (or too low). Stay focused. Find a support group.

Start. And don't look back.

CHAPTER 13

MY STORY

Now that the book has almost come to an end, I want to share my story with you: from beginning to end. Maybe, it will help you on your journey of weight loss. My story is not unique (there are many similar stories out there); it is not dramatic (you can always find more drama in life…). But what makes it beautiful is that it is my story.

You see, when I started off on my weight loss journey, many years ago, I was a very chubby teenager with many insecurities that felt like the biggest problem in the world. I was so focused on my problems that when I think about it now, I wonder how I even survived. Certainly, I was depressed and anxious most of the time.

My weight loss journey started with the idea that my extra pounds are the problem. I thought that when these pounds "melt off" I will no longer feel insecure or unhappy. However, when they did go away (for a couple of weeks or even months), my happiness levels did not rise. Sure, I felt happy for a moment or two, but this euphoria ended pretty soon and a new fear came up: I was afraid that the weight would come back. And it always did.

In pursuit of happiness (losing weight), I engaged in numerous weight loss programs. Some were more effective, others — not at all. Yet, each of these initiatives taught me something new. I tried keto dieting, being vegetarian, fasting, and numerous other approaches that were bound to bring me one step closer to my ultimate goal. They did, but always temporarily. At one point, about ten years into my weight loss journey, I realized that something was deeply flawed in my search. I was fighting myself vs. embracing myself. This is exactly why I undertook therapy. I decided to turn inward and explore why my efforts were not leading to any lasting results. These endeavors helped me to come up with a philosophy of my own. Eventually, I developed my own, unique plan (something that I hope you will do as well, using the knowledge and insight offered in this book and beyond it). I adapted this plan to my needs; I made it flexible. Quite soon I got the feeling that I was on the right path. Things finally felt right to me.

I no longer felt like I was conflicting with myself. The inner conflict started to dissolve. One of the traps that I fell into entails believing that when I found the "right path," the inner conflict would dissolve overnight. However, this was impossible. Only now I understand this. Since the inner conflict did not emerge overnight, it is unlikely that it can go away in a day or two. This process could take a substantial amount of time, so be prepared to do the hard work.

However, the good news is that as you move along the path of truth and integrity, your inner core is strengthened. This can be paralleled to regularly exercising in the gym. Your muscles gain strength, you gain stamina, and can exercise for longer periods of time, handling more pressure, more weight, etc.

CHAPTER 14

TRACK YOUR PROGRESS

Finally, I suggest that you track your progress on a weekly basis and write a summary of all that you have achieved or failed to achieve. This means having a set of criteria that you use to judge your progress. These measures could include the number of pounds lost (or gained). Also, you should keep a record of how well you have managed to follow through with your plan (or failed to do so). I suggest that you set a 90 percent mark for yourself. If you manage to stick to your plan 90 percent of the time, you are doing good. We are all human and sometimes fail to fulfill our plans/schedules; so do not be too rough on yourself. As for some other measures that you could use to track your progress, you can rely on smartphone applications in order to record how much water you drink and to set reminders for when to go to bed and when to get up. Having a stable schedule often works to your advantage.

One of the mistakes that I did when I embarked on my weight loss journey is that I did not track my progress as regularly as I should have. In fact, I would either check my outcomes too often or not at all. Thus, I suggest that you set a certain plan for yourself, such as checking your weight on a weekly basis and tracking how well you followed through with your plan. You could also record body measures (e.g., measuring your waist, thighs).

It is so crucial to track your progress because this way, you will see how your hard work is paying off. However, it is also important not to become overly focused on the final outcome and to enjoy the process. Remember, this is not a sprint. Here, in this book, we are talking about a life-long process of self-care. One that will last as long as you live. This is not some radical program that you have to stick to for a month or two and then drop it. It is something that you should integrate into your life and stick to it — forever.

These are self-care tips that will help you to stay healthy, fit, and happy for a long time. And, as we all know, in a healthy body there is a healthy mind. This is exactly why I suggest that you focus on several realms (not just the body). A holistic approach will take you farther than you have imagined. You will not only start loving your body, while making it more beautiful and healthier on a daily basis, but you are bound to feel greater satisfaction and happiness each and every day.

EPILOGUE

The main aim of this book is to show you that there is so much more to weigh loss than simply losing weight. We are complicated beings, with multiple needs and inner processes. Each of these processes has a tremendous impact on our bodies: how we feel, what we feel, and how we look (at the end of the day). With this said, it is highly important to be very attentive to your needs and to listen to yourself. This is not easy. It might take you many years and tremendous effort to learn to hear yourself (your heart, your spirit, and your body). But, it is well worth it. Dieting and exercising — all this should stem from your inner core. When you tap into your own needs, wishes, and aspirations, there is no longer a dilemma hanging over your head, leaving you full of doubt as to which path to take.

This book provides a series of tips that will "help you" to "hear" yourself better. What is more, a general list of tips is given that might help you to start walking down the path of a more fulfilling relationship with yourself (body included). If you are battling your extra weight, you will either come to accept this weight as normal and acceptable, or you will find ways (exercise, relaxation techniques, and a comfortable, healthy diet) that will help you to lose weight smoothly and without abusing your body.

Because, in the end…

Weight loss should never be about self-abuse.

It is always about self-love.